Shutting Doors

Sofia discovers resilience, kindness, and healthy choices during her grandmother's cancer journey

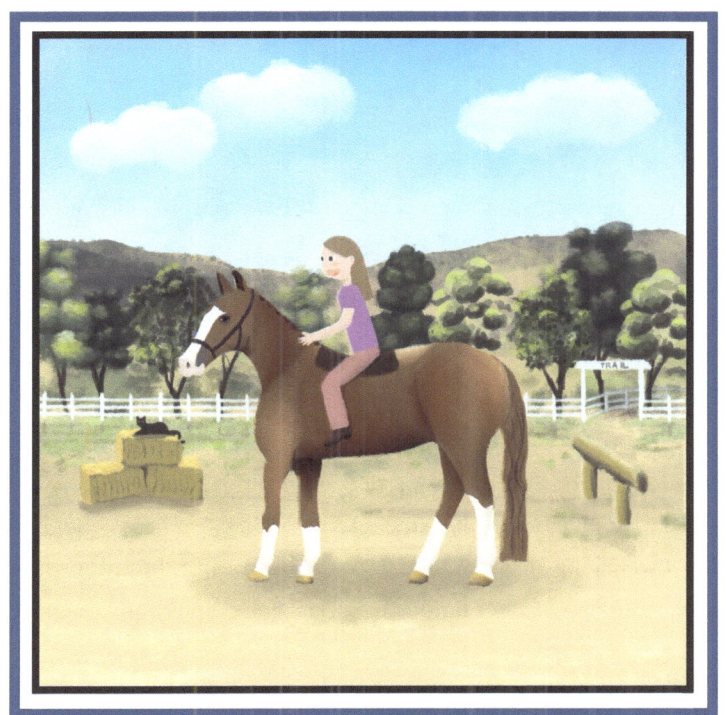

By Leslie O'Brien Sanders

Illustrated by Michael J. O'Brien

Copyright ©2025 by Leslie O'Brien Sanders
Published by Wolff Wellness Solutions LLC

Hardcover ISBN: 979-8-9933046-0-1
Softcover ISBN: 979-8-9933046-1-8
E Book ISBN: 979-8-9933046-2-5

All rights reserved.

No portion of this book may be reproduced in any form without written permission from the publisher or author, except as permitted by U.S. copyright law.

This publication is designed to provide accurate and authoritative information in regard to the subject matter covered. It is sold with the understanding that neither the author nor the publisher is engaged in rendering legal, investment, accounting or other professional services. While the publisher and author have used their best efforts in preparing this book, they make no representations or warranties with respect to the accuracy or completeness of the contents of this book and specifically disclaim any implied warranties of merchantability or fitness for a particular purpose. No warranty may be created or extended by sales representatives or written sales materials. The advice and strategies contained herein may not be suitable for your situation. You should consult with a professional when appropriate. Neither the publisher nor the author shall be liable for any loss of profit or any other commercial damages, including but not limited to special, incidental, consequential, personal, or other damages.

Illustrations by Michael J. O'Brien
Edited by Sue Copsey

1st edition 2025

Contents

Sofia's Rainbow 1

The Long Drive 3

Not Pouring, Just Drizzling 5

Thanksgiving Lessons 7

Warriors and Wigs 8

Touching the Bumpy Bump 11

Pieces of a Puzzle 15

Shutting Doors 16

The Monster Door 19

Finding Peace 21

Moving Matters 23

Kind Feels Good 25

Sleep is a Superpower	26
The Summer of Strength	29
Growing Through the Seasons	31
Dancing in the Rain	33
Living with Love	34
Glossary	36
Summary	37
Acknowledgements	38
Acknowledgements	39
About the Author	40
About the Illustrator	41

Dedication

Dedicated with endless love to my wonderful grandchildren who brighten every chapter of my life.

Jack & Dane
Myles & Sofia
Tayden & Elijah
Bryce & Zane
Everleigh & Easton

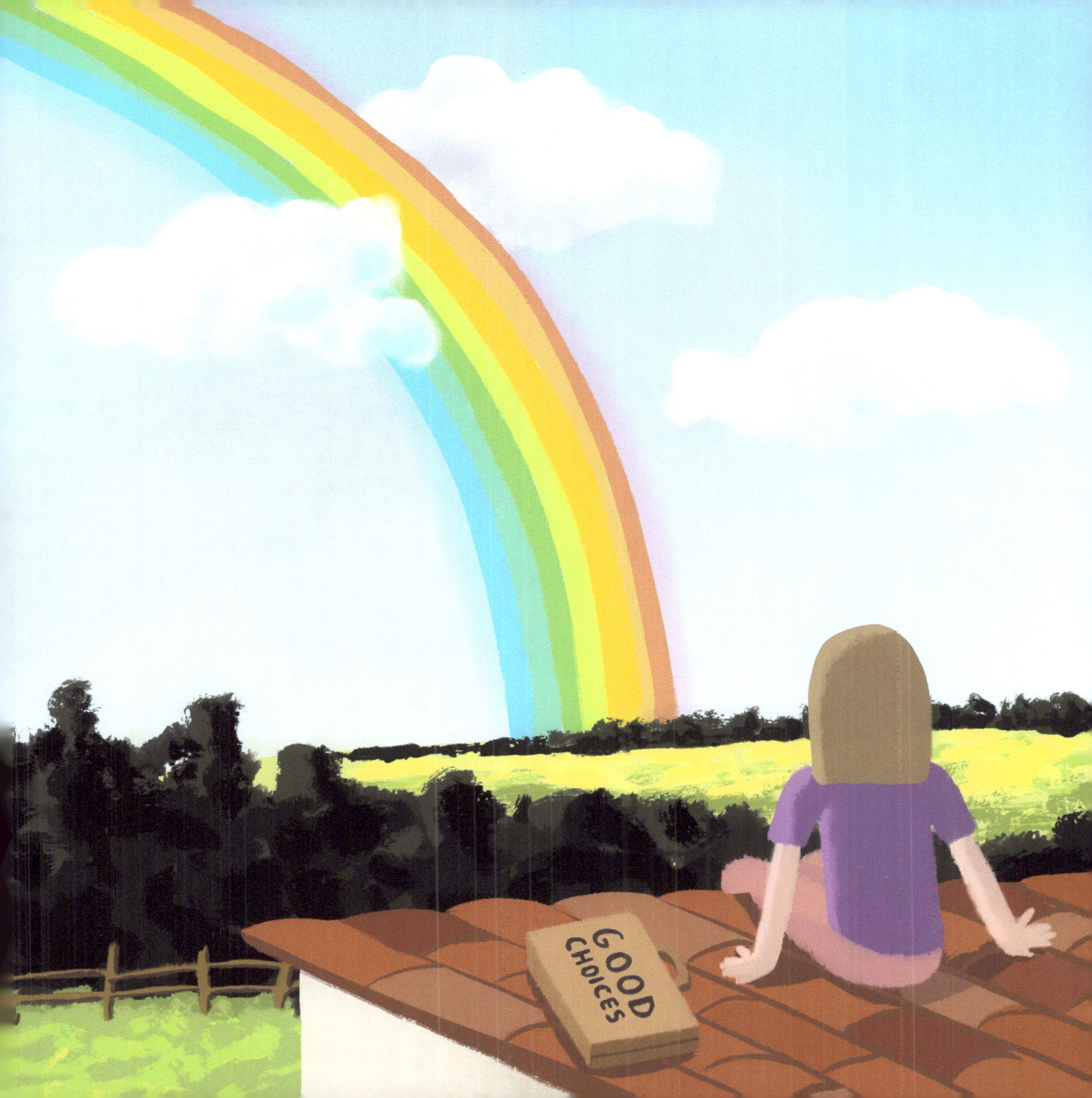

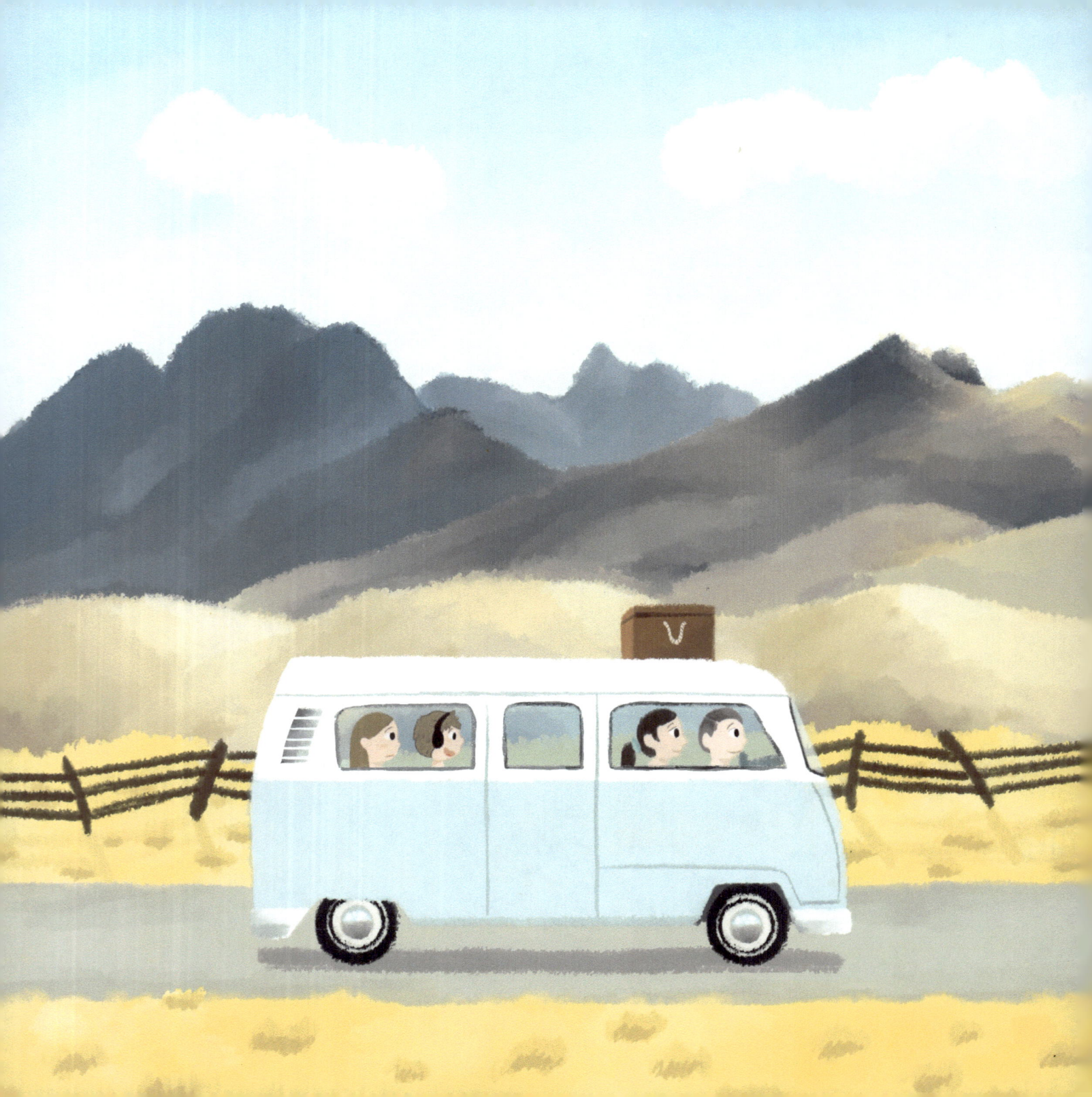

The Long Drive

Sofia squirmed in her seat and put down her tablet. They were taking her older brother Myles to camp, and the ride felt endless. Mom and Uncle Chris were in the front, talking quietly.

Myles was excited. He had his headphones on and was bouncing his legs. But Sofia's thoughts were elsewhere.

If Lita was in the car, she thought, *she'd be reading me my dragon chapter books.* (Lita was short for *Abuelita,* which is Spanish for "grandmother.") After all, Sofia was in Texas, and that meant special time with Lita. Being with Lita was her happy place. She liked hearing her grandmother say, "You make my heart smile."

"Why isn't Lita taking us to camp?" Sofia asked, looking at her mom's reflection in the rearview mirror.

Mom's face tightened for just a second.

Uncle Chris cleared his throat. "Lita just found out she has an illness called cancer."

Had she heard Uncle Chris correctly? Sofia's heart sank. Lita always said, "When it rains, it pours." Did this mean it was going to pour? Was something bad going to happen to Lita?

When they dropped Myles off, camp was buzzing with excitement, but Sofia felt a knot of worry.

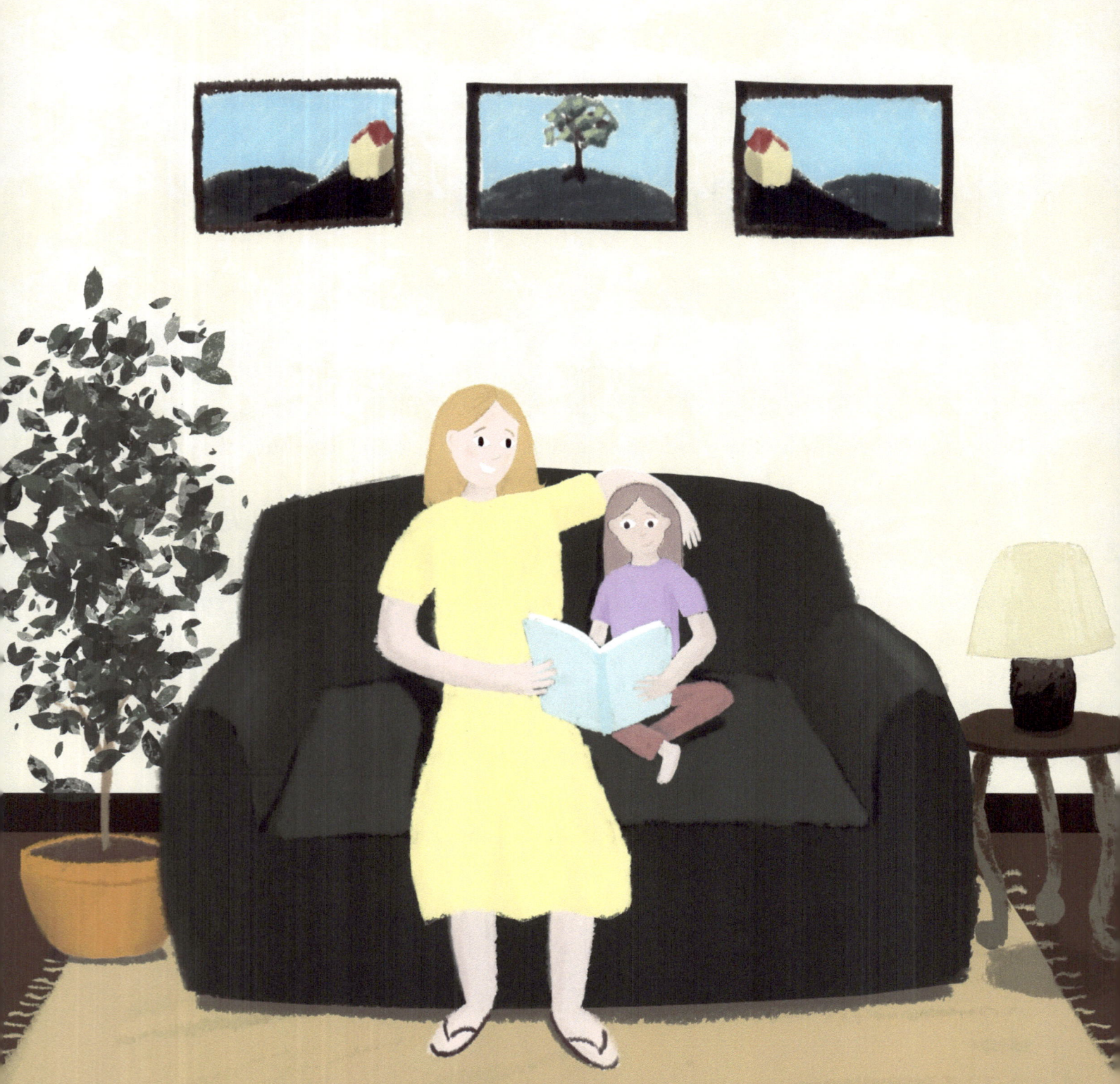

Not Pouring, Just Drizzling

The drive from camp back to Lita's house was quieter. Sofia stared out the window, still thinking about what Uncle Chris had said.

Back at Lita's, she was greeted with a great big warm, squishy hug. Sofia giggled. *This is what love feels like.*

Lita ran her a bubbly bath and read her dragon chapter books at bedtime. As they snuggled together, the fear Sofia had felt in the car began to fade. Maybe it wouldn't pour after all.

For the next two weeks in Texas, Sofia tried not to think about Lita's illness, but sometimes she caught her grandmother deep in thought. And Grandpa did the cooking more often than he used to. (Spaghetti, again.)

Being at Lita's felt *almost* the same, but something was a little off—just enough for Sofia to notice.

Thoughts of Lita's cancer kept sneaking back. "Cancer is bad," Myles had told her.

Back home, she vowed to talk to Lita every time she called. *I'm glad she doesn't talk about cancer*, Sofia thought.

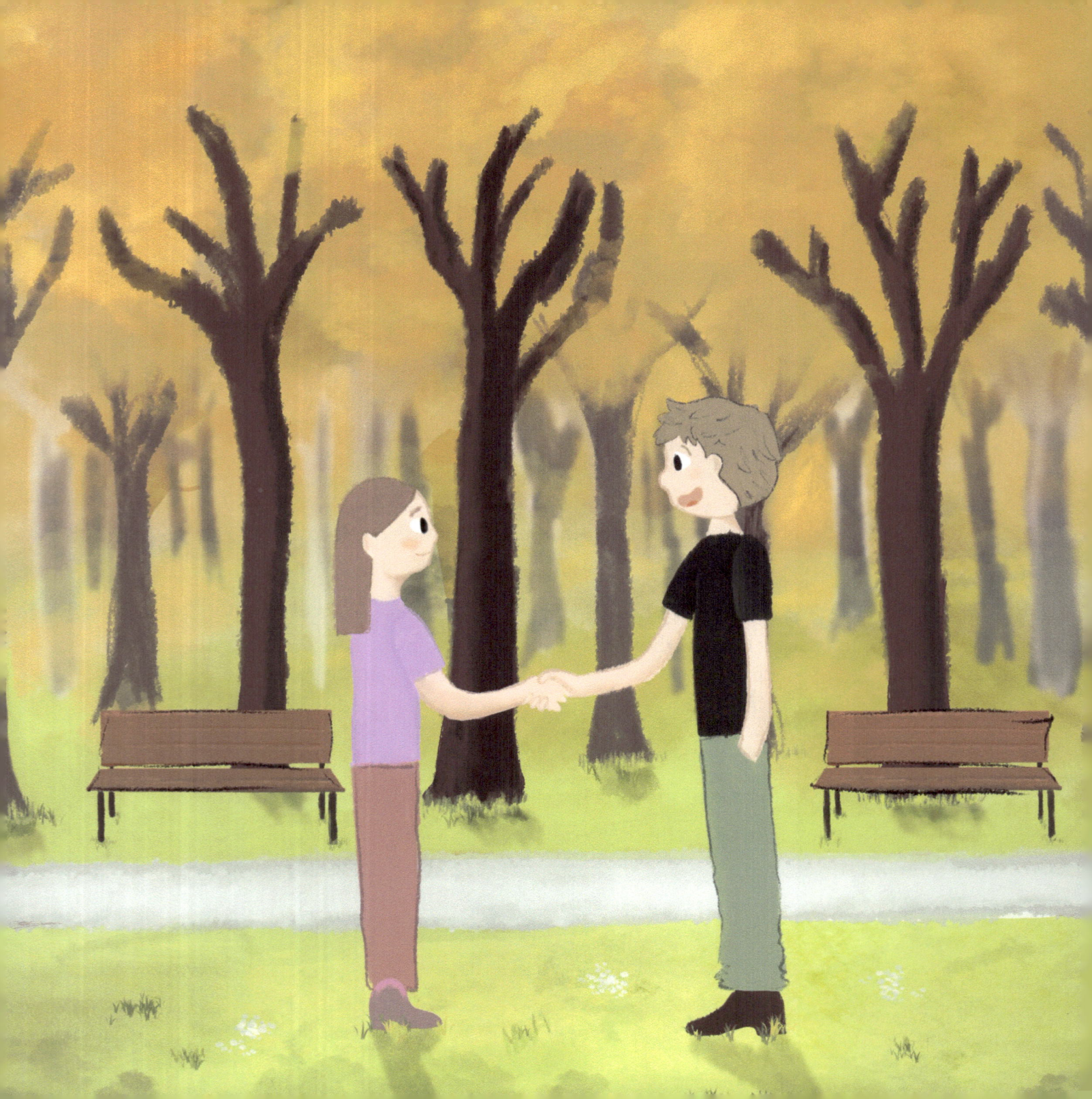

Thanksgiving Lessons

A few months later, Sofia was reminded about Lita's cancer.

"It's important we spend Thanksgiving with Lita," Mom announced.

The family packed up the car, and even Tenaya, their dog, joined them for the trip to Texas.

They spent time camping by the river with their older cousins, Jack and Dane. Sofia tried to focus on the fun—swinging from the rope, swimming, kayaking, playing with the dogs. But every now and then, she saw Myles watching Lita with a worried face.

Lita was taking lots of naps, and she was losing her hair. It reminded Sofia of Tenaya—hair everywhere!

"Sofia," Myles said, "I'm proud of Lita. She's fighting as hard as she can. She's a warrior."

They made a pact to make sure Lita knew they were happy to be spending Thanksgiving with her.

Warriors and Wigs

"Lita *is* a warrior," Sofia told Myles. She didn't think it was fair that Lita had cancer, and yet her grandmother never complained.

Lita explained that she was being treated with strong drugs, and that this kind of treatment with chemicals was called chemotherapy. Each dose of drugs was called an "infusion."

Sofia felt sad. *Poor Lita. No wonder she's always tired and her hair's falling out.*

"Dragging her to the clinic is like trying to take a cat to a bath," Grandpa said. Sofia laughed a little. *I wonder if Mom says that about me on school days.*

During their visit, Lita took Sofia and Myles wig shopping with her. Wow! So many hairstyles lined up in endless rows—curly, straight, and spiky. Sofia giggled, *Snip, snip, snip—giving haircuts could be fun.* (Supervised by Lita, of course.)

Sofia liked a soft, long-haired wig. "Yuck," Myles said, choosing a fluffy one.

Lita laughed and chose a short one—it was stiff but practical, she said. "It's just hair," she added, walking out with all three wigs. But Sofia noticed how her grandmother's smile quickly disappeared.

She gave Lita a great big hug. "I love you, Lita," she said, and Lita's smile came back.

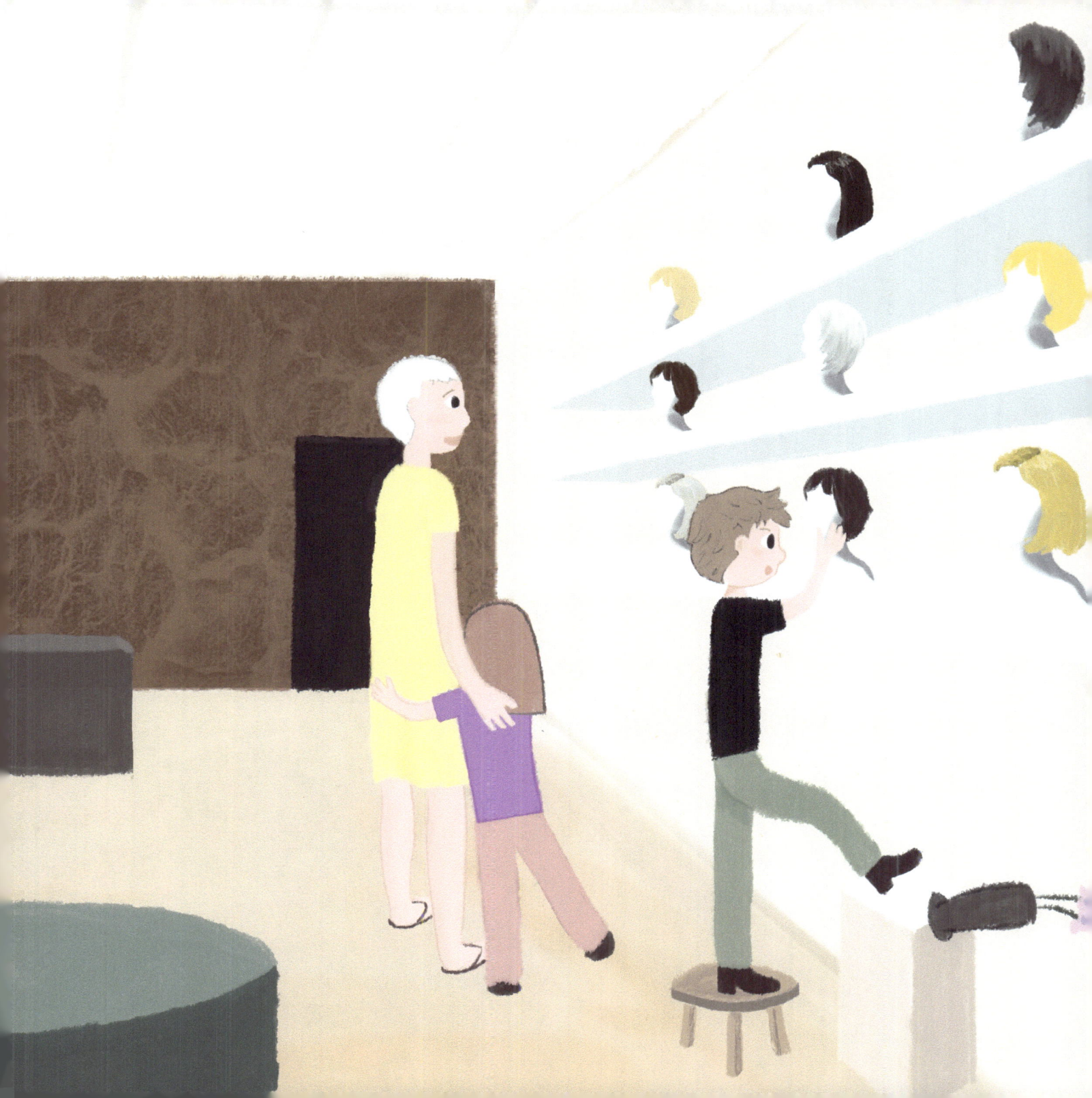

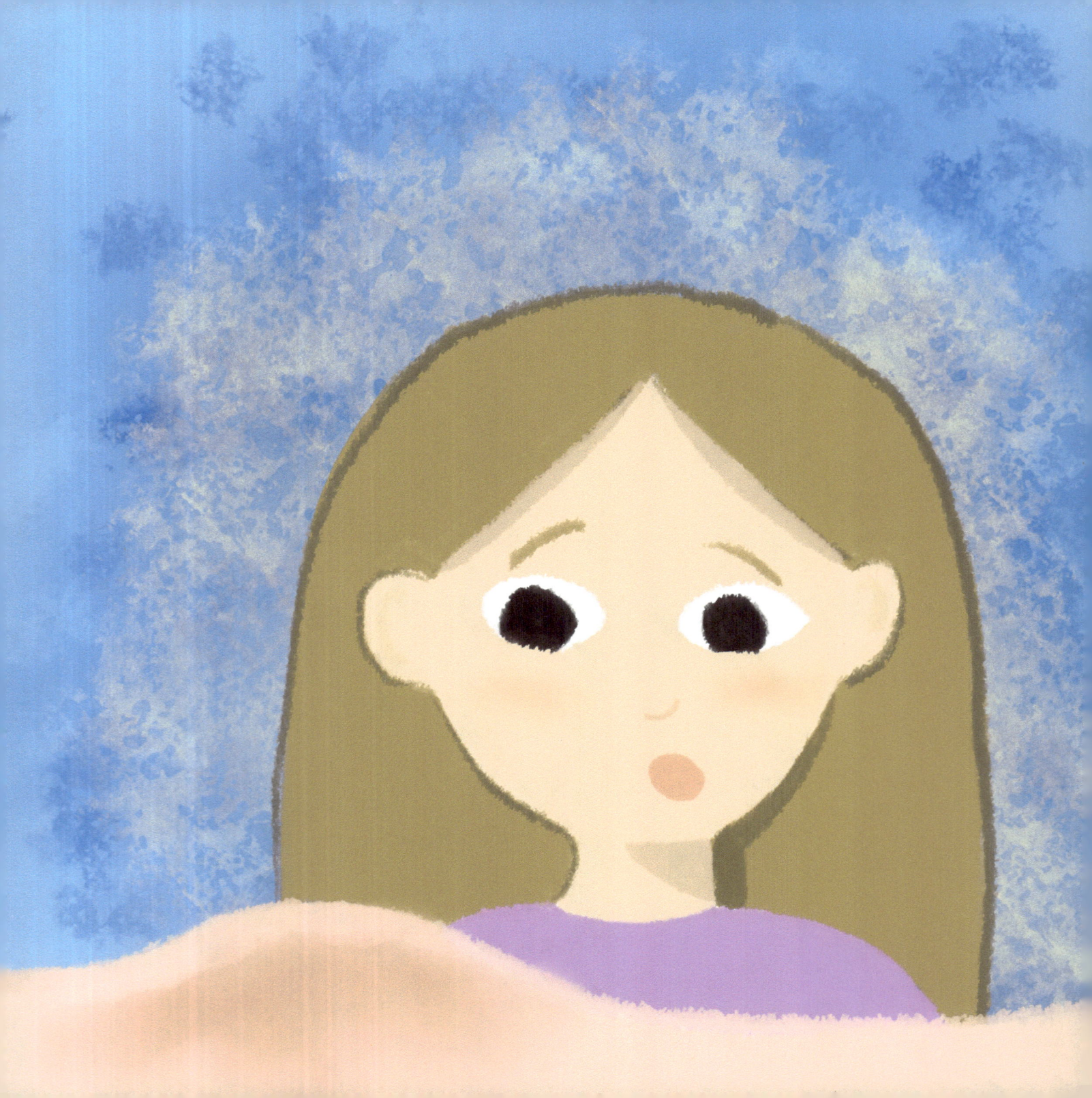

Touching the Bumpy Bump

Sofia was curious about cancer, and wanted to find out more about it. She learned that it was caused by a few abnormal cells growing out of control.

She knew that cells were like teeny tiny factories with BIG jobs. Cells kept all living things alive.

"Our bodies have trillions of cells," Myles told her.

Sofia asked if she could touch the bumpy bump on Lita's chest. It was the special spot, called a port where the medicine could go straight into her blood—like a superhero's power port.

Myles wasn't interested in touching it. Lita had wrinkled her nose when Sofia asked. Sofia thought it was kind of neat, rubbing her fingers on the bumpy bump.

It had been a special Thanksgiving after all. Back home, Sofia looked forward to video calls with Lita.

But she decided, *We won't talk about cancer anymore.*

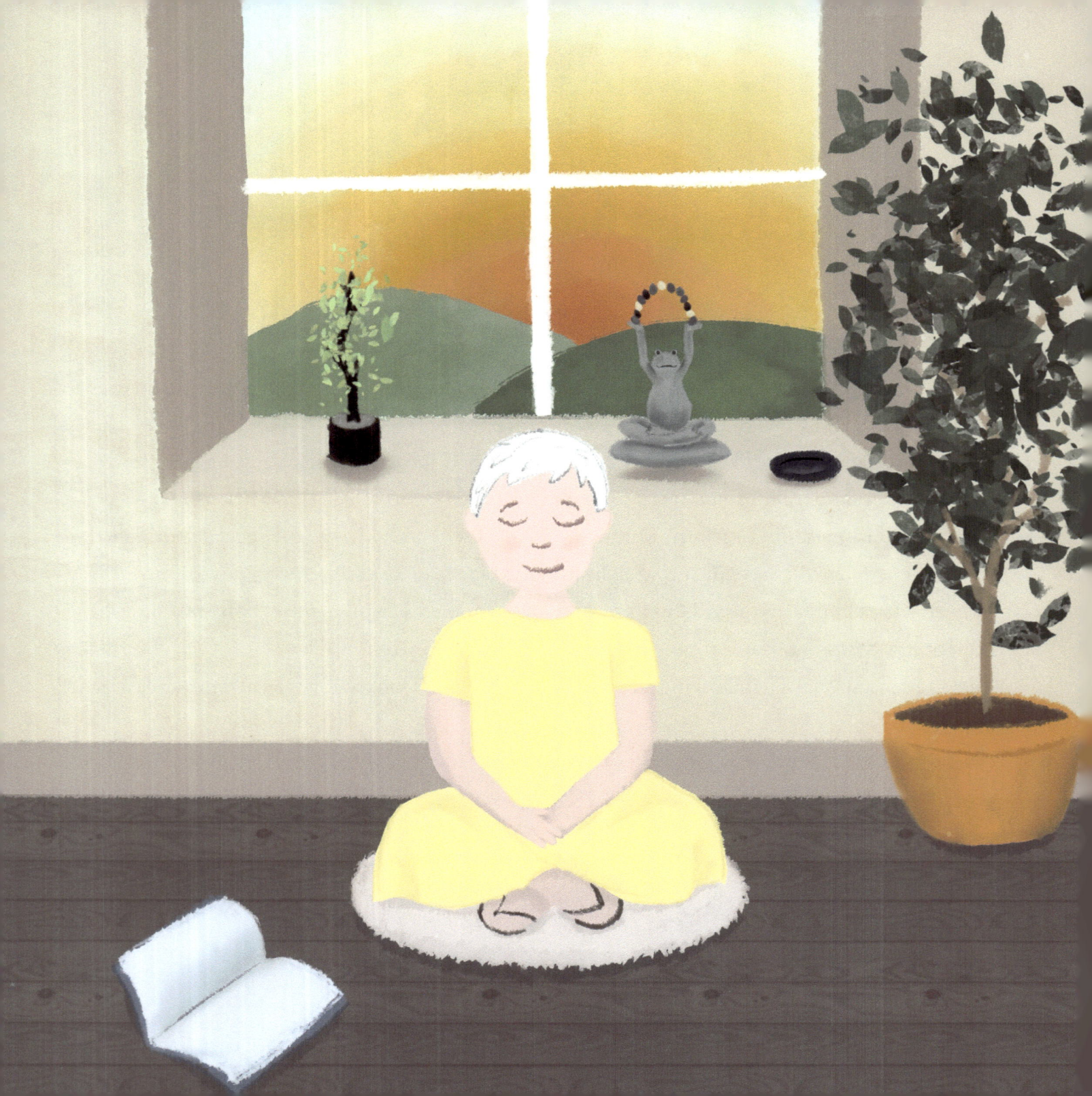

A Coach Steps In

At Christmas, they *did* talk about cancer—but Lita's words had changed. She told Sofia and Myles that she had a cancer coach now.

"She's teaching me a new way to look at things," Lita explained. "Positive thinking."

This sounded a lot like the growth mindset Sofia learned about in school—the one that turned *I can't* into *I can't yet*. It had inspired her to practice more and work harder.

"I'm not fighting cancer," Lita said. "I'm surrendering to healing."

The knot in Sofia's stomach came back. She didn't understand. Warriors fought, didn't they?

"Like a warrior in a battle, surrendering to healing also needs action, courage, and strength," Lita explained. "It creates space to focus on what really matters."

At first, Sofia didn't know what to think. But when she saw the change in Lita, she hoped that surrendering was okay—and that maybe Lita wouldn't have cancer anymore.

But Sofia continued to worry about Lita's new mindset.

I choose to think of Lita as a warrior.

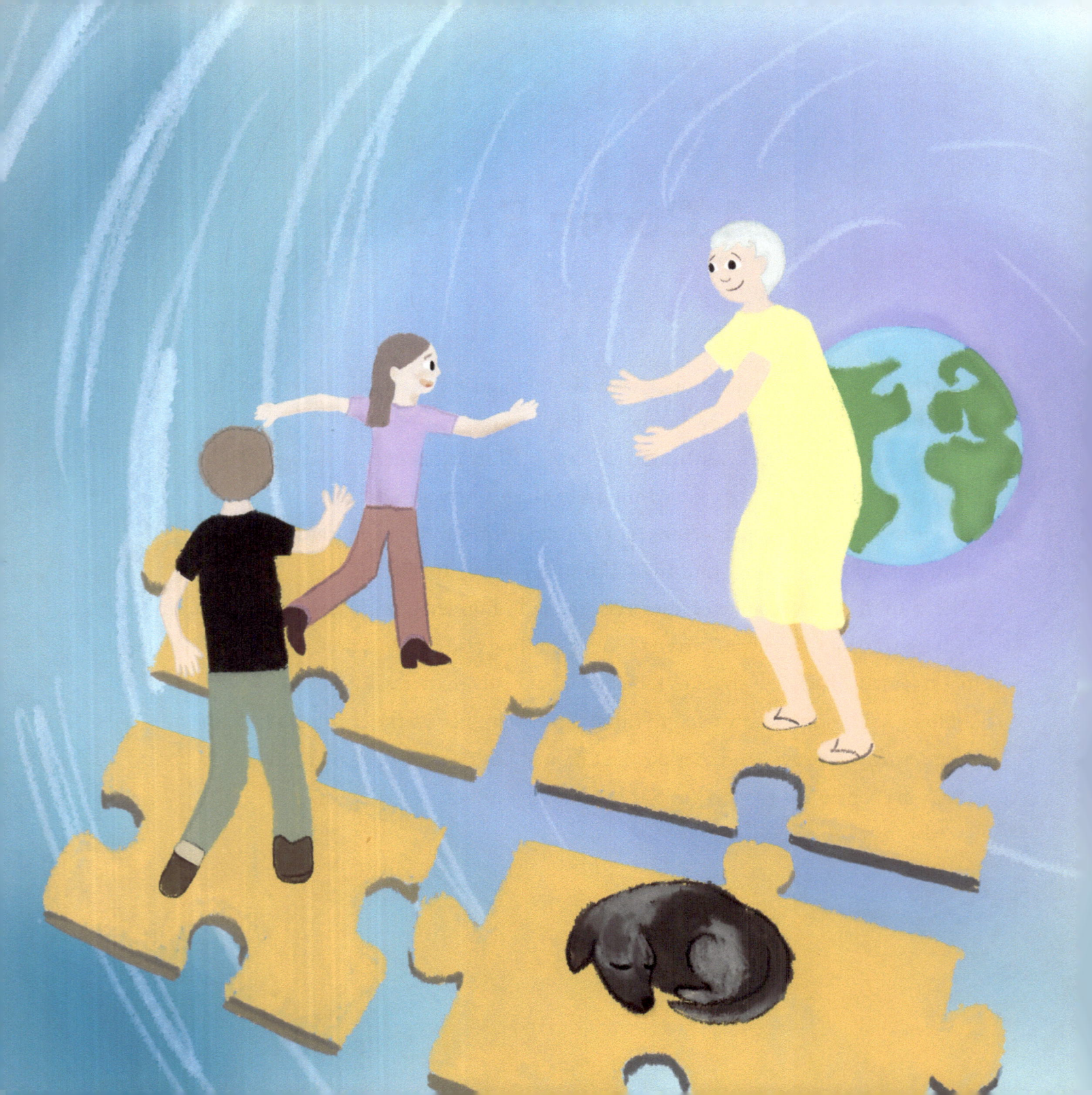

Pieces of a Puzzle

With the start of the new year, Sofia's warrior had more to say about what she was learning from cancer and her coach.

"It is important to love yourself," she said one day. "All the support and prayers, from family, friends—even people I've never met—touched my heart so deeply. They made me realize my life truly means something,"

I knew Lita was special, Sofia thought. *How come she didn't know it?*

"Loving ourselves and understanding our importance on this earth makes life easier. We all have a purpose," Lita explained.

Sofia thought of a puzzle—every piece mattered. Puzzles couldn't be finished without all the pieces in the right place.

I am important too! Each piece is as important as the others.

Sofia wasn't sure she knew what loving herself looked like. But Lita gently said it could start with small choices.

Shutting Doors

"Small choices and actions have important consequences," Lita told Sofia.

Lita's lessons began to flow naturally into their lives. She taught Sofia and Myles about what her coach called "shutting doors", which meant getting rid of bad habits that could lead to illness like cancer.

She decided that her kids and grandkids should start learning to keep these cancer doors shut tightly. "Now is the time to start healthy life-long habits like eating well, drinking plenty of water, finding peace, staying active, and getting enough sleep."

Sofia pictured good dragons guarding each doorway, keeping out cancer cells that tried to grow uncontrollably. They must be powerful fire dragons, she decided.

"Shutting doors is one way to love yourself," Lita said. "Each door you keep shut honors your body. That's a big part of loving yourself."

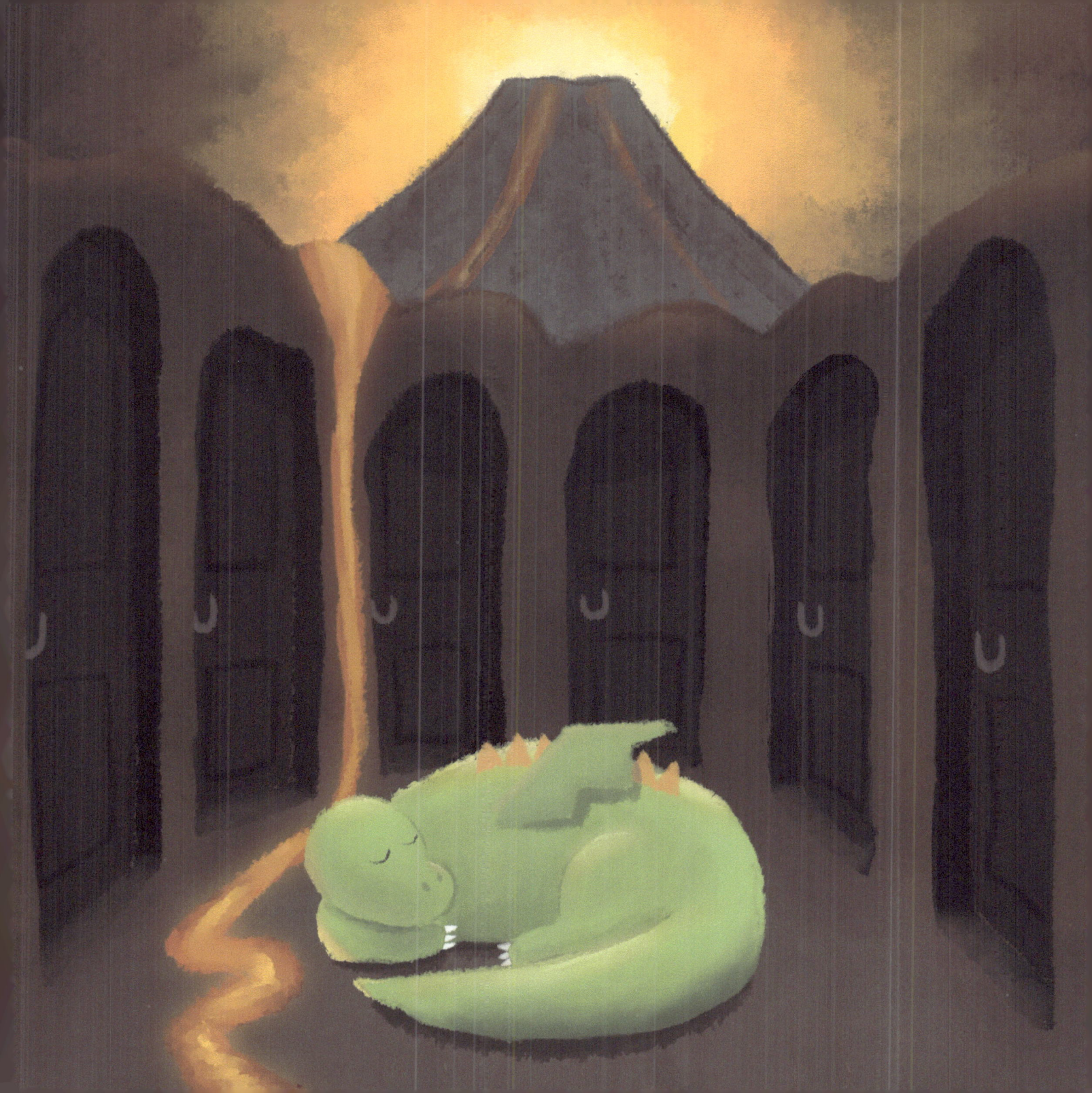

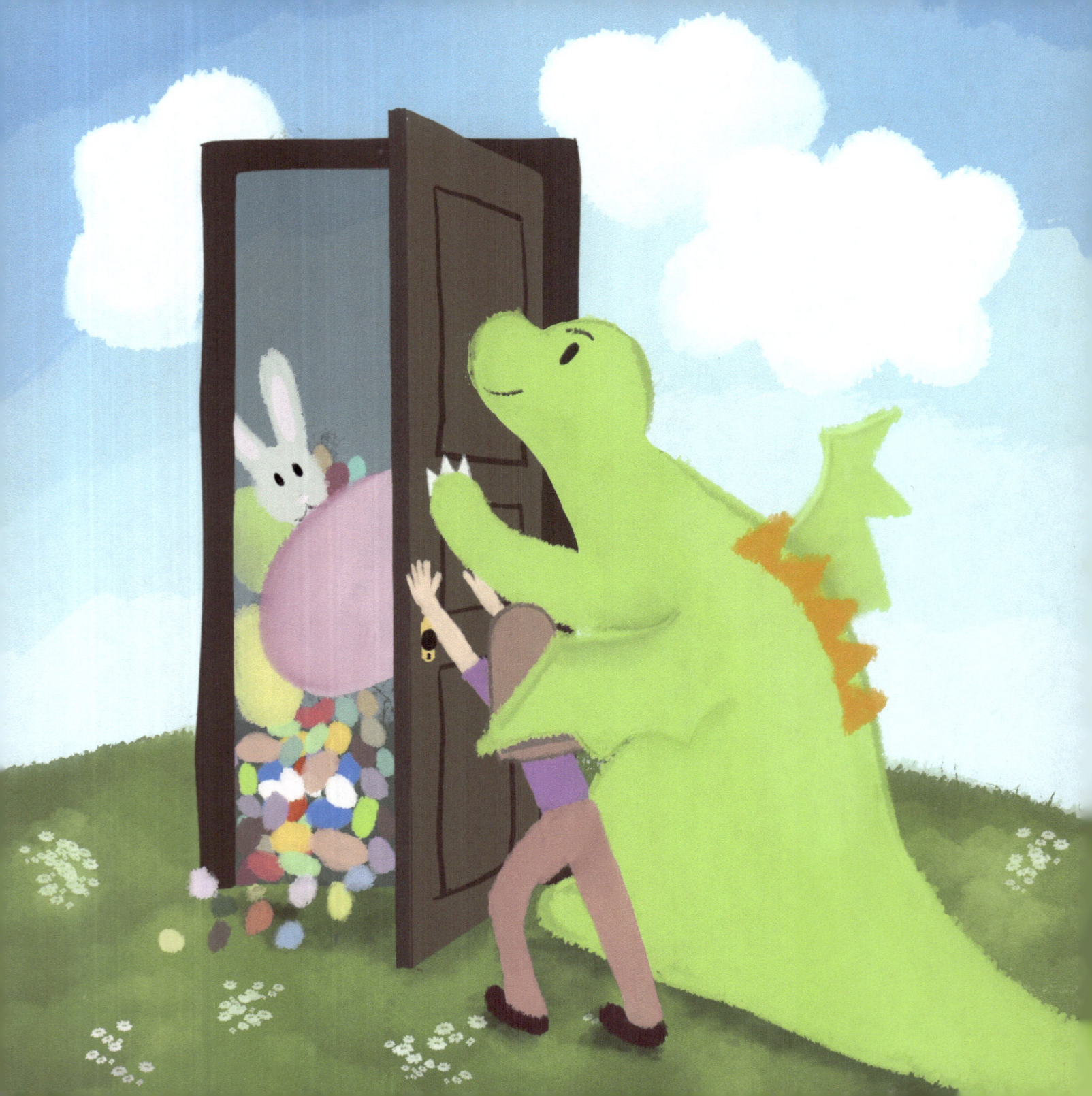

The Monster Door

Sofia thought that eating food that's good for you must be the Monster Door. She might have to do some talking with that dragon!

Lita talked a lot about the importance of eating more plants like fruits and vegetables in many colors. "Eating the rainbow," she called it.

Sofia did the math and thought eating three to five different colors a day might be hard. There were plenty of nice types of fruit, but she could count on one hand the vegetables she liked.

Lita stressed the importance of eating less sugar.

Just great, Sofia thought. Cutting back on candy, cookies, and ice cream. *Is that really necessary?*

Lita added that drinking lots of water to stay hydrated went along with good eating habits.

Shutting this HUGE door was going to be a chore.

Easter was coming soon. Surely, the Easter Bunny would still leave chocolate eggs? Wouldn't he?

Sofia would have to wait to find out.

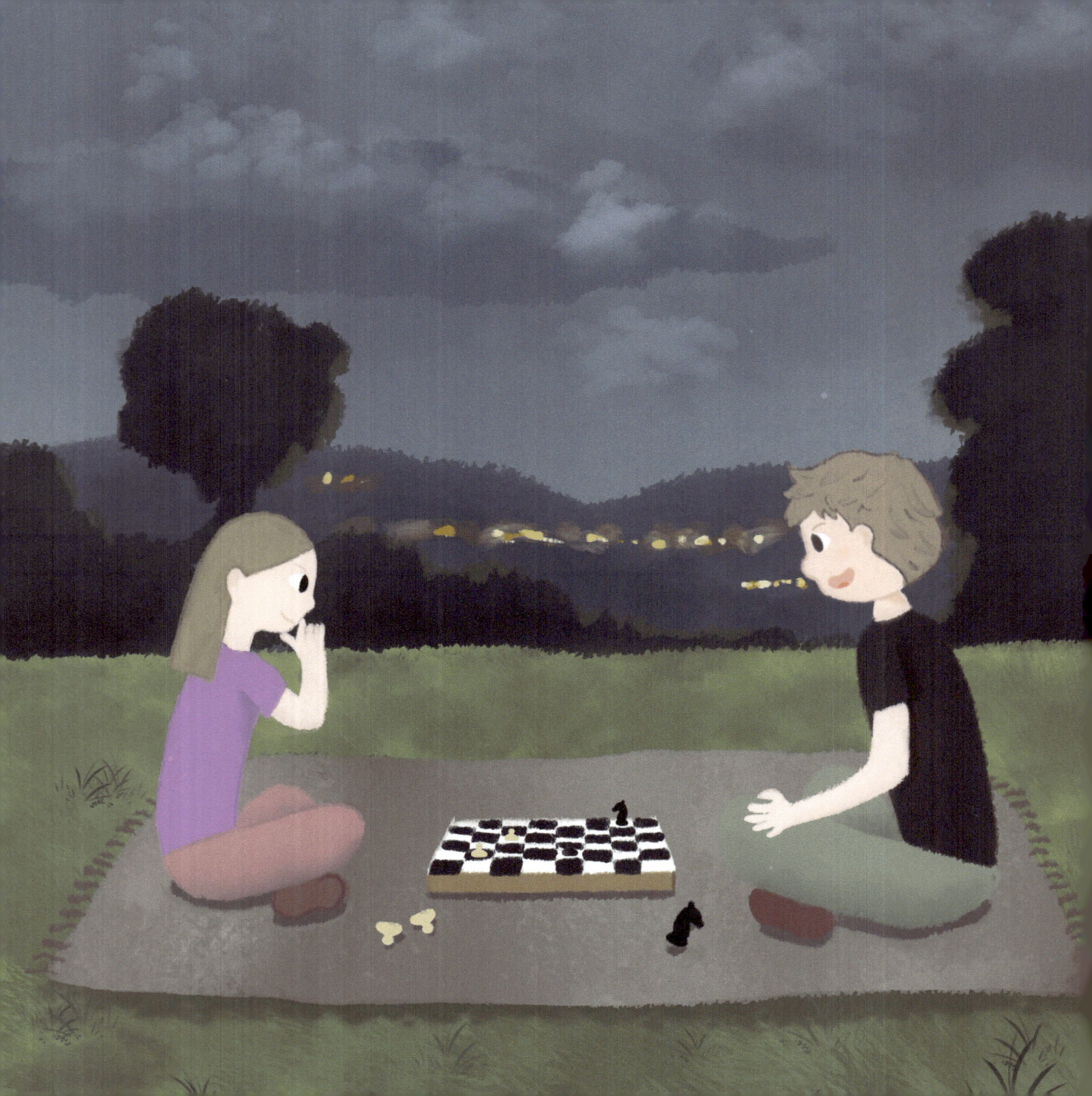

Finding Peace

Finding peace and stillness was part of Lita's day. She called this "being mindful." Lita meditated, sitting quietly, focusing on her breathing. A calming voice or quiet music helped her. She allowed thoughts to come and go, drifting by like clouds.

Sofia placed a hand on her own stomach, feeling it rise and fall. Playing with her breath and noticing the movement was fun.

Lita also made time for prayer—God was her source of strength and help—and she read stories about other people who had faced challenges in their lives.

Lita wrote down daily thoughts, reasons to be grateful, and celebrations. Sofia was surprised that even little things, like a phone call with one of her grandkids, made it into Lita's journal.

When I go to college, I'm going to call Lita every day, just like my cousin Jack does.

"Finding activities that make me feel good brings me joy, and helps me understand that I can accept life with cancer," Lita said.

Sofia kept only good thoughts in her head—there just wasn't room for bad ones. That's what helped her feel calm, just like Lita.

Playing chess with Myles feels like a mindful moment, thought Sofia. *I sit still, my eyes focused on the board, thinking carefully with each move—trying to outsmart him and keep my pieces safe.*

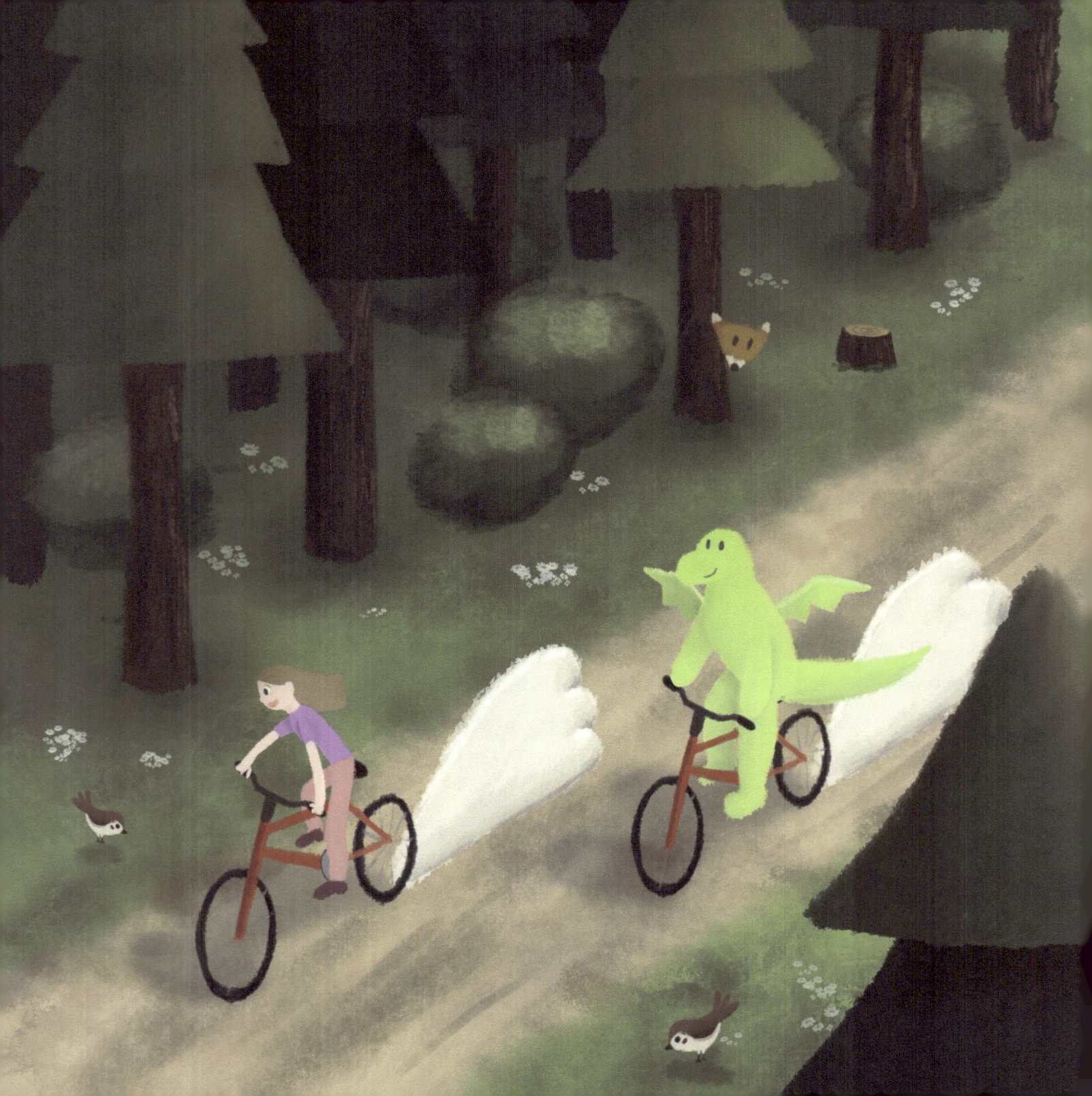

Moving Matters

Sofia lost count of how many doors she was supposed to keep shut. She wanted to make Lita happy, but shutting doors was becoming hard work.

To her delight, the next dragon Lita talked about was fun—moving and staying active.

Easy-peasy, Sofia thought.

She loved being outdoors: riding her bike, kayaking, hiking, and swimming in the summer; skiing and ice skating in the winter.

But I spend a lot of time indoors playing on my tablet, she admitted to herself.

Sofia liked trying to keep up with Mom during online exercise classes, especially when Lita joined in too. Lita also enjoyed yin yoga—slow, gentle stretches that made her feel peaceful.

Even Sofia's tías (Spanish for aunts) were big fans of yoga. It felt like something special they all shared.

Lita also walks, Sofia thought. *Surrendering to healing does require action.*

Myles admitted that video games were keeping him indoors, and that now spring was here, he should be outside.

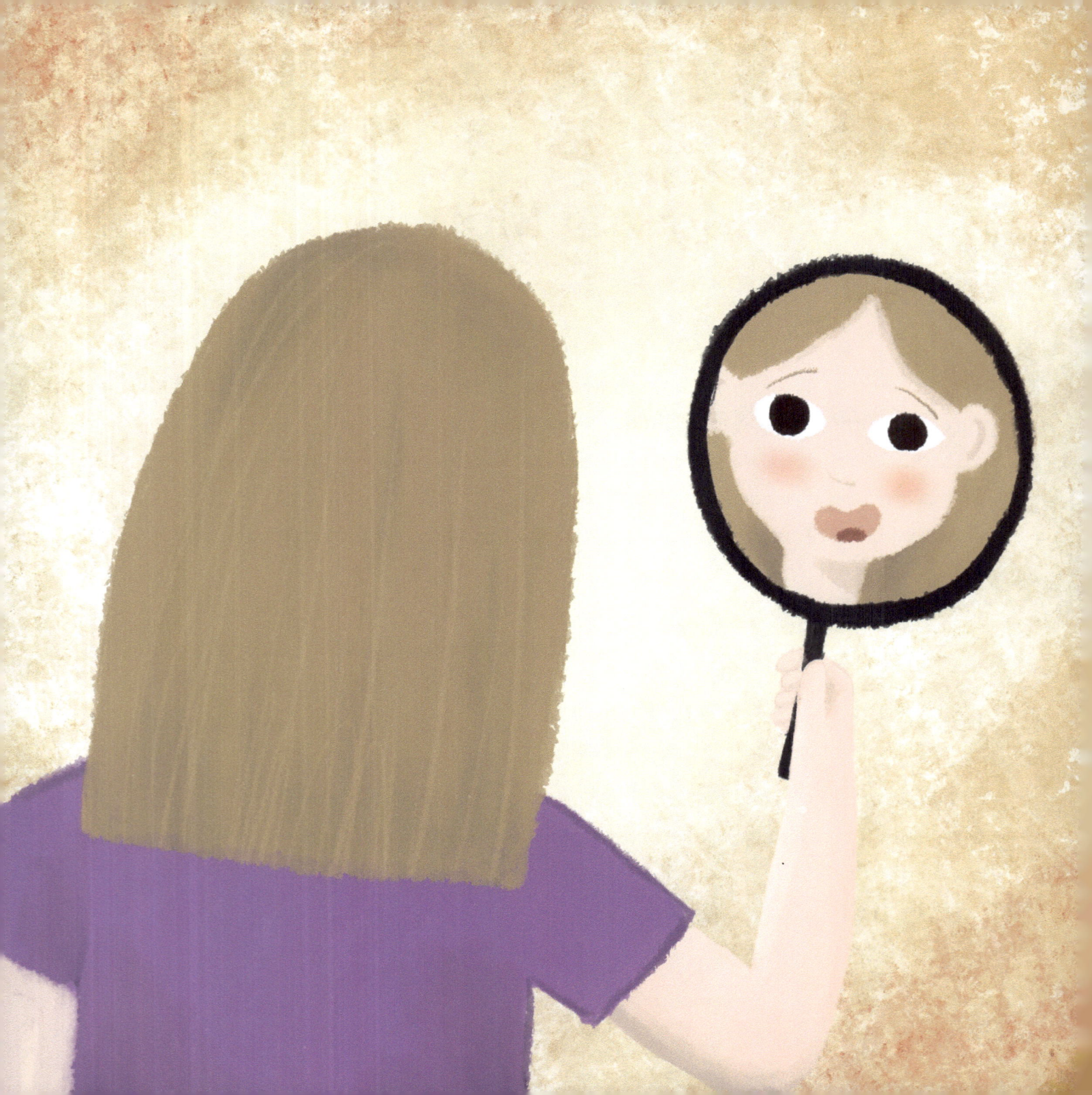

Kind Feels Good

One day, Sofia's teacher told Mom that Sofia was kind and accepting of others.

Loving myself must make it easier to appreciate others, Sofia thought.

She realized that just smiling at someone created a connection that felt good inside.

I'm starting to like this feeling, she thought.

Loving yourself mattered. Being kind and connecting with others brought joy.

Proudly, she shared this new door with Lita and Myles.

It might be my imagination, Sofia thought, *but I think Myles is trying to be kinder, especially to Lita. Does he know something I don't?*

With summer—and another visit to Texas—around the corner, Sofia would get to show Lita her progress.

Sleep is a Superpower

In June, the school year finished, and Sofia was looking forward to camp. She and Myles were in different tribes, which meant they wouldn't be cheering for each other.

Let the games begin!

Thinking about camp was her new favorite way to fall asleep. *It's more fun than counting sheep!* But sometimes, she worried just a little bit.

What will my bunkmates be like?

Will we be besties?

What will my horse be like?

Myles, however, was confident he'd get a great horse, and wasn't worried about his bunkmates.

Sofia knew that a good night's sleep was one more cancer door shut. And it was also a good way to start the day. Lita always said, "The early bird catches the worm."

Sofia's excitement grew day by day. She'd worked hard to stay healthy, and now it was time to enjoy summer.

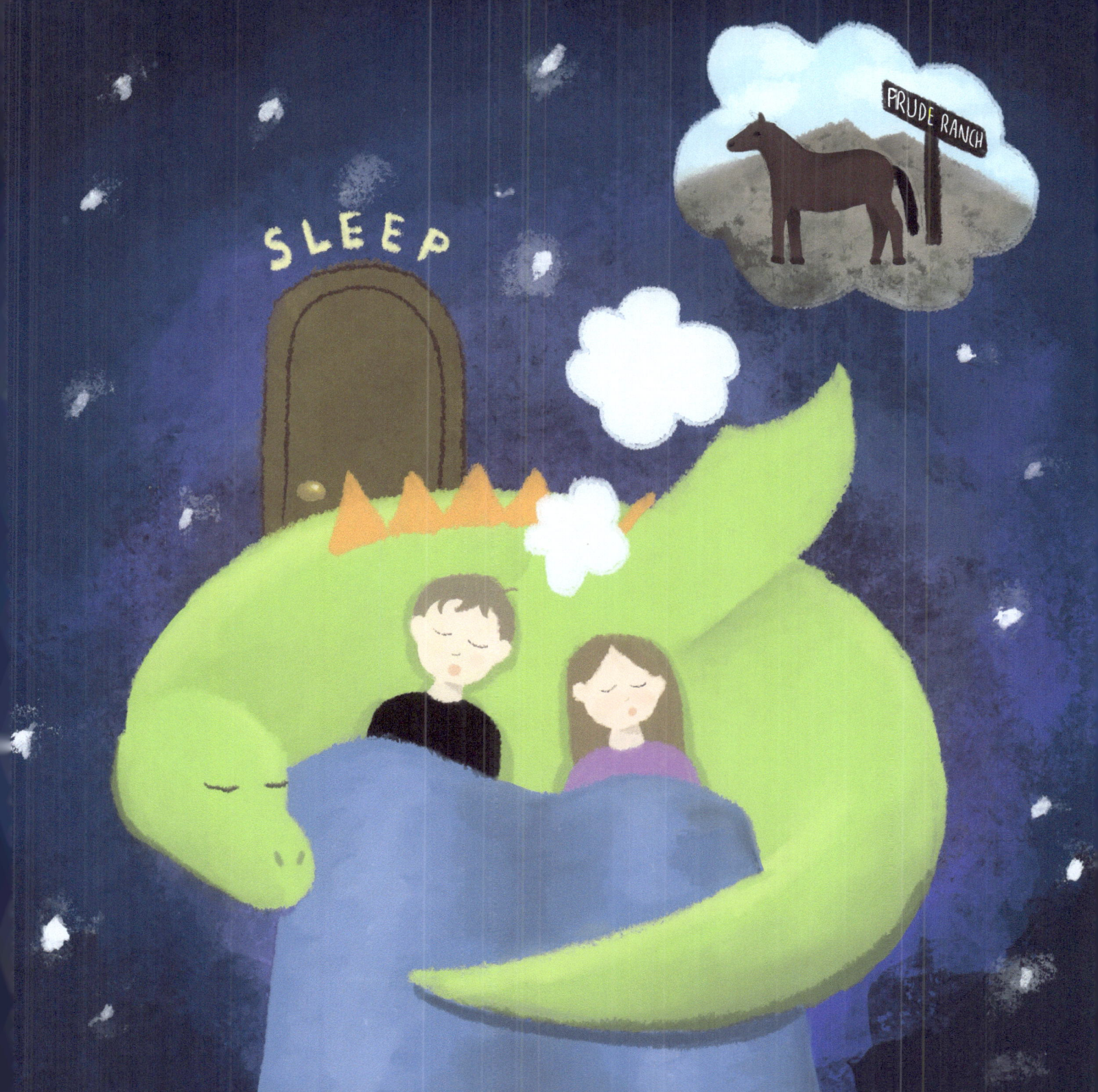

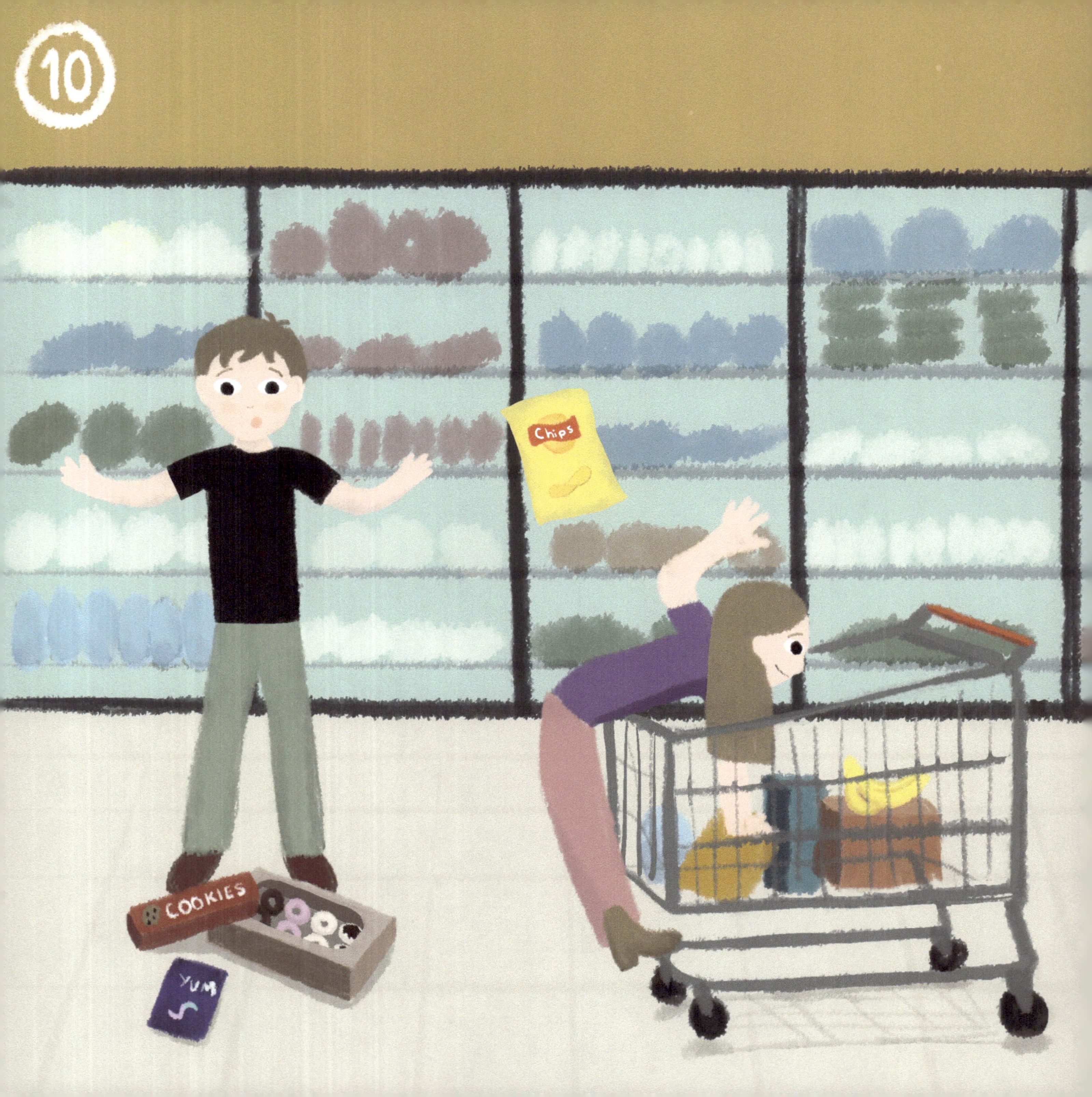

The Summer of Strength

July came, and Sofia and Myles went off to camp. Sofia was nervous about her first rodeo, but Lita reminded her she could do difficult things. When she won Most Improved Rider, she felt a burst of pride.

Back at Lita's house, life had changed. Lita had taught them about eating the rainbow—fruits and vegetables of all colors—and the dangers of sugar, and now Sofia and Myles were label detectives at the store, hunting for hidden sugars.

Water bottles and healthy snacks were a regular part of their routine.

Quiet now meant being mindful—an opportunity to be present and grateful.

Sofia and Myles stayed off their electronics for longer. Swim goggles in hand, they raced each other to the pool.

Splash! "I win again!" Myles proudly yelled. "You cheated again!" Sofia responded.

Connecting with others—and being nicer to Myles and her parents—brought more joy and smiles into Sofia's life. *It would be nice if Myles would try it too.*

Going to bed early when the sun was still up wasn't so easy to do in the summertime.

Loving yourself isn't easy to understand, Sofia reflected. *But somehow, it works.*

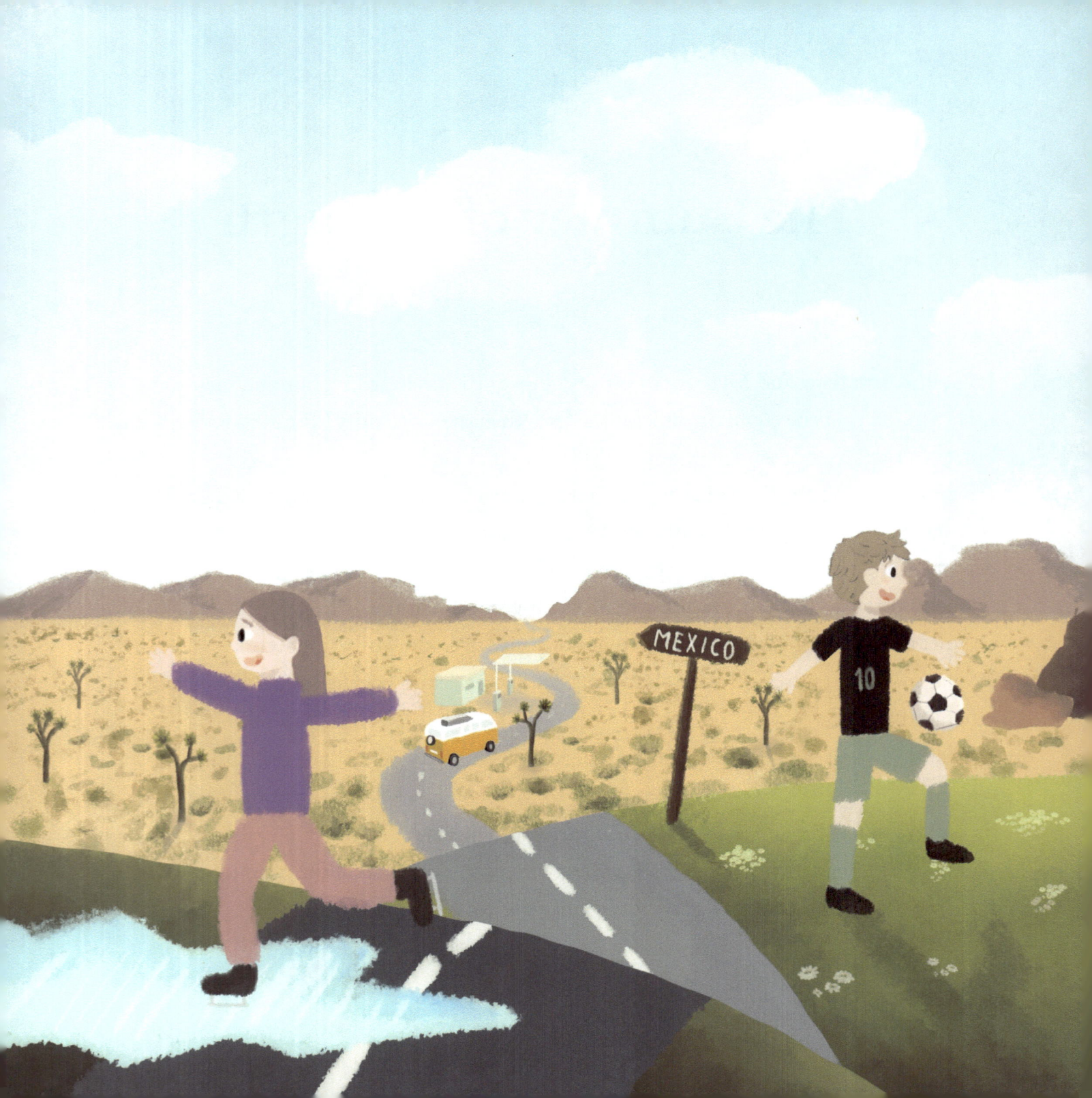

Growing Through the Seasons

Summer was over, and Sofia was in second grade.

She had learned some important life lessons from Lita's cancer journey. Shutting doors by adopting healthy life habits was a way to lessen the chances of getting cancer.

Her brother didn't talk about cancer doors, but Sofia noticed he was getting better at shutting them—even if he, too, still struggled with that Monster Door.

Sofia wasn't trying to make new friends, but she still tried to be kind. *Everyone has a role to play*, she thought, *like those pieces in a big, important puzzle.*

In the fall, Sofia watched Myles play soccer, then when winter came, she went ice skating and skiing. In spring, she and Myles hiked in the mountains and swam in the hot springs.

The family took a trip to Mexico for spring break, and Tenaya came too.

Second grade hadn't been so bad. Sofia had stopped saying, "It doesn't matter," and "I don't care." Adding a positive mindset to her toolbox made her feel more confident.

I wonder if Lita will drive us to camp this year. Sofia's excitement grew each day—another summer was just around the corner.

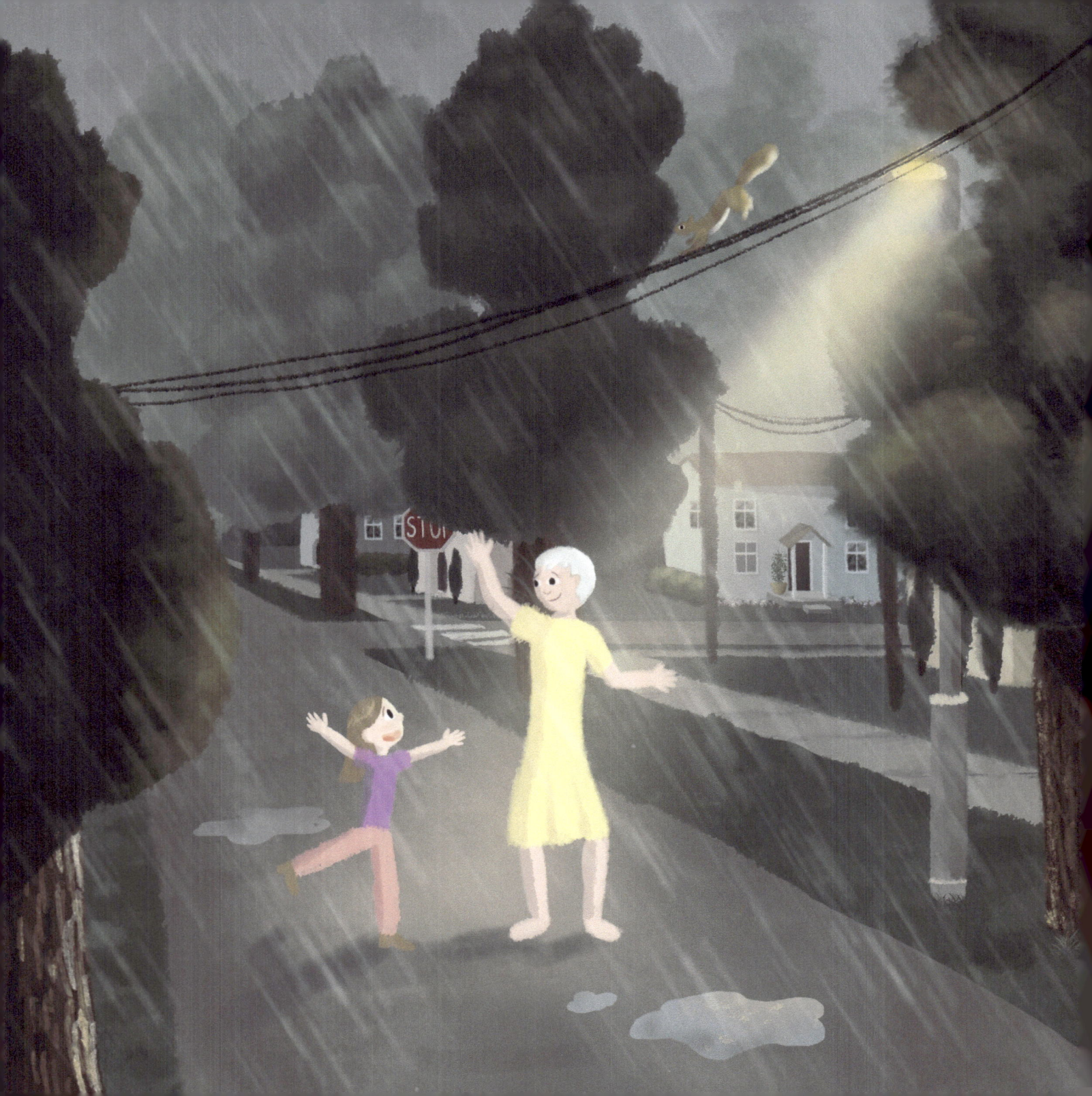

Dancing in the Rain

Summer finally came. This time, Lita, Mom, and Uncle Chris drove them to camp!

Sofia and Myles were excited to get there—and just as happy to be picked up.

"I'm exhausted!" they said before falling asleep on the drive home.

Lita was still laughing and still snuggling Sofia at bedtime. Her hair had grown back—it was silver now—but she was proud of it. Lita liked to say she had earned that gray hair.

Funny, Sofia thought. Lita always said, "When it rains, it pours." But now Sofia knew it doesn't always pour—and sometimes, you can dance in the rain.

Watching Lita travel, cook, visit with family and friends, and even make a quilt with cousin Dane during her two-year cancer journey made Sofia imagine Lita dancing in the rain.

Of course, Lita was also busy keeping doors shut. "Cancer's not stopping me from living my best life," she said.

Sofia and Myles both felt proud. In Sofia's mind, Lita was dancing in the rain!

Living with Love

Sofia realized Lita's lessons weren't just about avoiding cancer—they were also about loving and living your best life.

Now, whenever Sofia thought of Lita, she thought of strength, love, and what Lita called "the power of a positive mindset." And she knew those lessons would last forever.

While snuggled up to Lita one night, Sofia silently promised to love herself, love life, find joy, do hard things, have a positive mindset, and keep "cancer doors shut."

Cancer became less scary the more Sofia understood it.

Lita's wisdom kept unfolding with the seasons.

Not every door was hard to close—some were surprisingly fun.

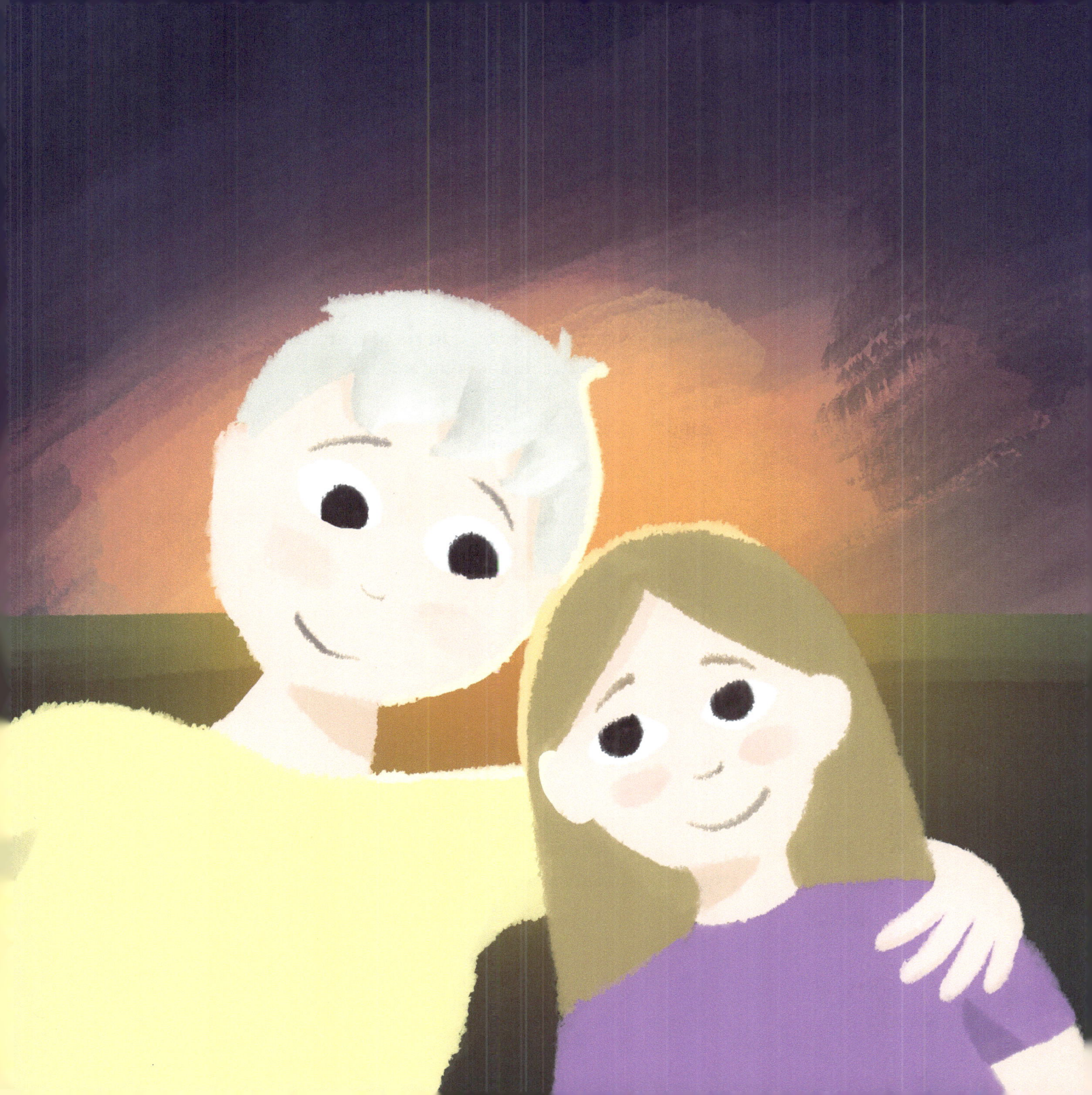

Glossary

CANCER - A type of sickness that involves the abnormal growth and copying of cells.

CHEMICALS - Water, liquid or gas that has specific features or characteristics we can use to identify it. Some chemicals are made by nature and some are made by people.

CHEMOTHERAPY - A combination of chemicals intended to help stop or lessen the growth of cancer cells.

CELLS - The building blocks of all living things. Cells are so small that you can't see them without a microscope.

HYDRATION – Having enough water in your body to stay healthy.

INFUSION THERAPY - A way of providing fluids or medication directly into a patient's bloodstream.

MINDFUL - Thoughtful attention.

PORT - A small implantable object that is placed under the skin and attached to a vein. It allows medical staff to get blood without having to use a needle and to deliver chemotherapy drugs or other fluids directly to a vein.

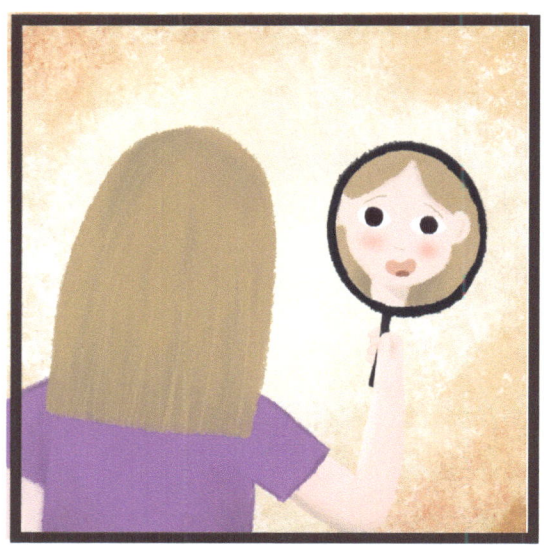

Sofia's Lessons

Find Joy

Have a Positive Mindset

Keep Cancer Doors Shut

Know You are Important

Love Life

Love Yourself

You Can do Hard Things

Cancer Doors

Eat Well

Drink Water

Find Peace (Happy Place)

Stay Active

Be Kind (Connect with Others)

Get Good Sleep

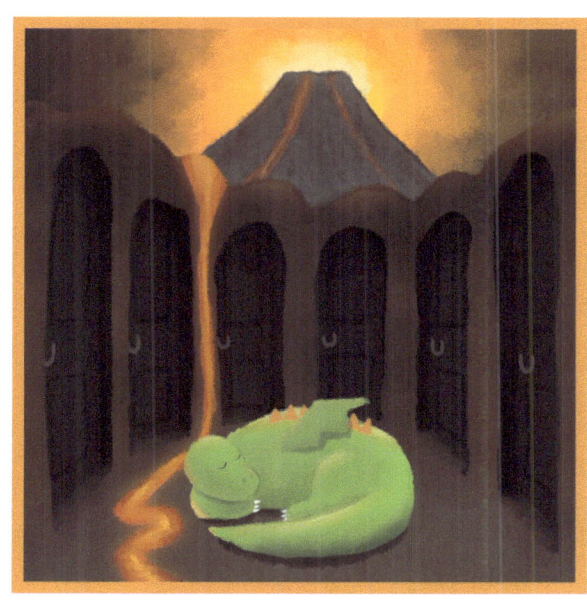

Acknowledgements

With a heart full of gratitude and love for my MAGNIFICENT support team empowering me on this journey.

My husband, children, siblings, and grandchildren
My wonderful friends—the fiercest prayer warriors ever!

With endless gratitude and admiration to my extraordinary care team.

Dr. Christopher Braden & Staff – Texas Oncology – New Braunfels

Dr. Juan Diocares – Texas Digestive Disease Consultants – New Braunfels

Dr. Ryan Huey & Staff – MD Anderson Cancer Center – Houston

Rachele Jaeger & Trainers – The Vfit Studio

Trisha Knudson – Red Bird Acupuncture & Eastern Medicine

Elissa Lueckemeyer RDN, LD – Food 4 Success

Leslie Nance, CHCC, CHN – Any Stage Cancer/The Cancer Boss Program

Ronda Sober – Soul Shine Apothecary and Wellness

Acknowledgements

A special shoutout to those behind the scenes who helped me look my best, when I didn't feel my best.

Danny Nguyen & Jenny Tran – Best Nails & Spa

Natasha Peterson – Lily Lane Hair Studio

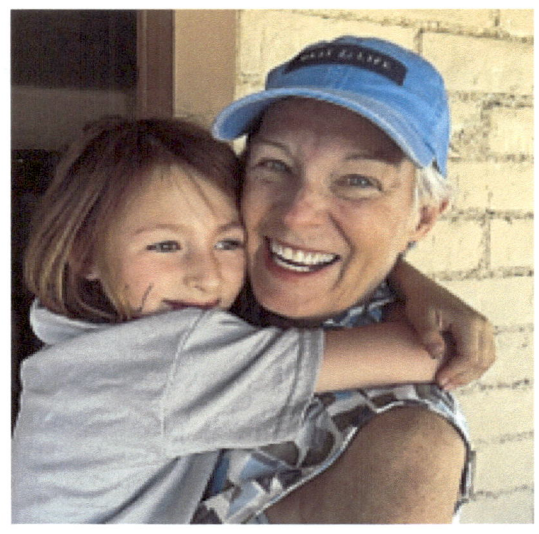

About the Author

Leslie O'Brien Sanders grew up in Panama, where a vibrant cultural background shaped her open-minded worldview. A former first-grade and bilingual Spanish teacher with a Master's in Curriculum Development, her love of children's literature inspired her to write her own. After a stage four pancreatic cancer diagnosis, Leslie found strength in her support network, care team, and cancer coach. Her journey now fuels her mission to share lessons on healthy living and the power of mindset through stories inspired by her granddaughter, Sofia.

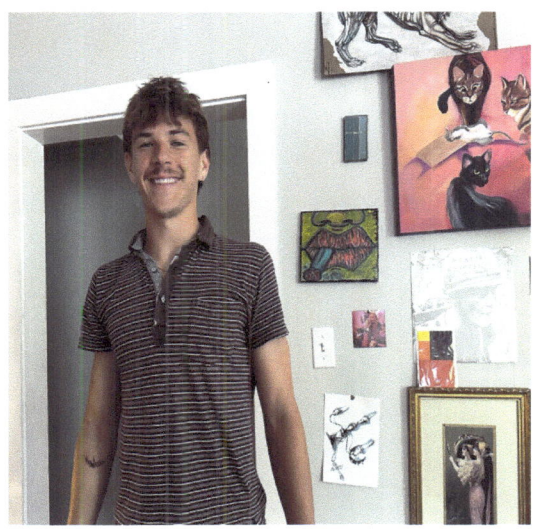

About the Illustrator

Michael J. O'Brien was born and raised in Italy, where a rich cultural heritage shaped his love for art. As a child, he combined his passion for soccer and art by making illustrations of his favorite soccer players. Today, he continues to pursue both soccer and art as a student athlete studying Graphic Design at the Savannah College of Art and Design.

www.ingramcontent.com/pod-product-compliance
Lightning Source LLC
Chambersburg PA
CBHW061156030426
42337CB00002B/27